YOUR KNOWLEDGE HAS VALUE

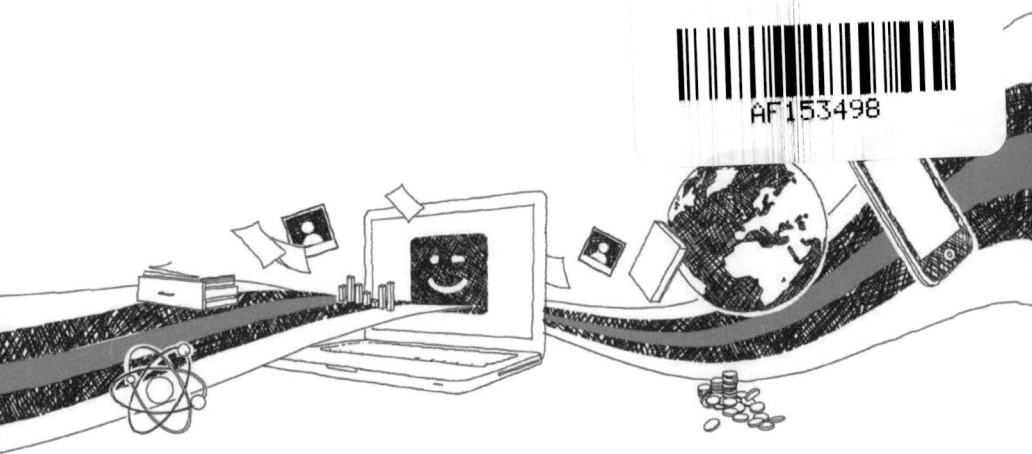
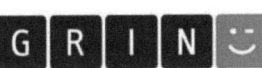

Usage of Vitamin D for viral infections with a focus on Covid-19 disease and the proposal of a study design

Felix Rubenbauer

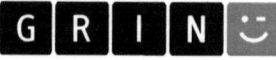

Bibliographic information published by the German National Library:

The German National Library lists this publication in the National Bibliography; detailed bibliographic data are available on the Internet at http://dnb.dnb.de.

ISBN: 9783346738349
This book is also available as an ebook.

© GRIN Publishing GmbH
Nymphenburger Straße 86
80636 München

Print and binding: Books on Demand GmbH, Norderstedt, Germany
Printed on acid-free paper from responsible sources.

The present work has been carefully prepared. Nevertheless, authors and publishers do not incur liability for the correctness of information, notes, links and advice as well as any printing errors.

GRIN web shop: https://www.grin.com/document/1281745

"Usage of Vitamin D for viral infections with a focus on Covid 19 disease and the proposal of a study design"

Submitted by: Felix Rubenbauer

Friedrich-Schiller-University Jena

EDU College of Medicine

Bachelor of Medicine

Submission date: 31.12.2021

Table of Contents

Abstract

In recent years, the popularity of vitamin D has risen in the alternative medicine spectrum as a "universal" substance for all sorts of diseases. Although many of the claims cannot be backed by scientific evidence, strong evidence still demonstrates the beneficial effects of vitamin D for treating various conditions that are not directly related to hypovitaminosis. Currently, there is evidence that demonstrates that the supplementation of vitamin D can prevent or relieve upper respiratory infections and endemic influenza. Additionally, herpesviruses are responsive to treatments that incorporate vitamin D, and antibody titers seem to be higher in individuals with higher vitamin D levels. For viral hepatitis, viral DNA load and seasonal fluctuating vitamin D levels seem to correlate with each other. Regarding Covid-19, there is a clear correlation between the disease's course and duration and vitamin D serum levels. However, it remains unclear whether low vitamin D levels can increase an individual's susceptibility to Covid-19 or whether Covid-19 causes low vitamin D levels. Furthermore, it is unclear whether a part of Covid-19's typical symptoms could be caused by a vitamin D deficiency. To uncover high-quality evidence regarding this topic, the author proposed a clinical trial to evaluate the effects of vitamin D supplementation on Covid-19 hospitalisation rates. The main outcome concerns the hospitalisation rates of intervention groups vs control groups regarding disease progression and the infectivity of cohort-isolated patients being secondary outcomes.

Introduction

Vitamin D has a primary role in the metabolism of calcium and, therefore, plays an important role in preventing rachitis in children and osteomalacia in adults. In recent years, researchers have investigated vitamin D's impact on the immune system and general health. A meta-analysis published by Zhang Fhang et al. in 2019 suggests that vitamin D supplementation could reduce cancer mortality by 15% (1). A randomised controlled trial that was conducted by Shirvani Kalajian et al. in 2019 could prove that the expression of certain immune-system-relevant genes changes under different levels of vitamin D (2).

Covid-19 is a disease caused by the SARS-CoV-2 virus, which has spread as a pandemic since spring 2020. At the time this paper was written, over 280 million people were infected, and 5.4 million had died as a result of contracting Covid-19 (December 2021, Johns Hopkins University). In mild and moderate cases, the disease presents with flu- or cold-like symptoms and can escalate in severe cases to ARDS and eventually cause death due to multi-organ failure. Since late 2020, vaccines that fight the SARS-CoV-2 infection have been made available. As several new virus variants that possess certain degrees of escape mutations have begun to spread, additional preventive measures are welcomed.

Regarding Covid-19, Pereira Damascena et al. proved in November 2020 that amongst hospitalised Covid-19 patients, the rate of vitamin D deficiency was 64% higher than in a mild case group (3). This finding suggests that vitamin D supplementation could benefit Covid-19 patients and potentially be used to treat other viral infections. The purpose of this paper is therefore to evaluate the effect of vitamin D as a cheap and widely available substance on prevention and therapy of common viral infections, the physiological backgrounds for the supposedly good efficacy in viral infections and the proposal of a trial design to improve knowledge about clinical implications of vitamin D application in Covid-19 patients.

Vitamin D

Vitamin D3 (cholecalciferol) is a fat-soluble steroid-style vitamin that regulates calcium, magnesium and phosphate homeostasis by upregulating intestinal calcium absorption. In vitamin-D-deficient individuals, the absorption of calcium can be reduced by up to 75%, which can cause rickets in children and osteomalacia in adult patients (4). The two major types of vitamin D are vitamin D2 (ergocalciferol) and vitamin D3 (cholecalciferol). Both have similar biochemical properties: ergocalciferol has a lower binding affinity to the vitamin D binding protein than cholecalciferol, and cholecalciferol is unable to bind to the vitamin D receptor without prior hydroxylation (5, 6).

Physiology

Cholecalciferol is produced by breaking up the B-ring of 7-dehydrocholesterol, which occurs when bare skin is radiated with UVB light from the sun. Ergocalciferol is mainly taken in with food. After synthesis, cholecalciferol is hydroxylated in the liver into 25-hydroxyvitamin D3 (25[OH]D) and subsequently in the kidneys into 1,25-dihydroxyvitamin D3 (1,25[OH]2D). The presence of this active form increases intestinal calcium absorption by activating the synthesis of the calcium-binding protein by binding to the vitamin D receptor and activating gene expression (7).

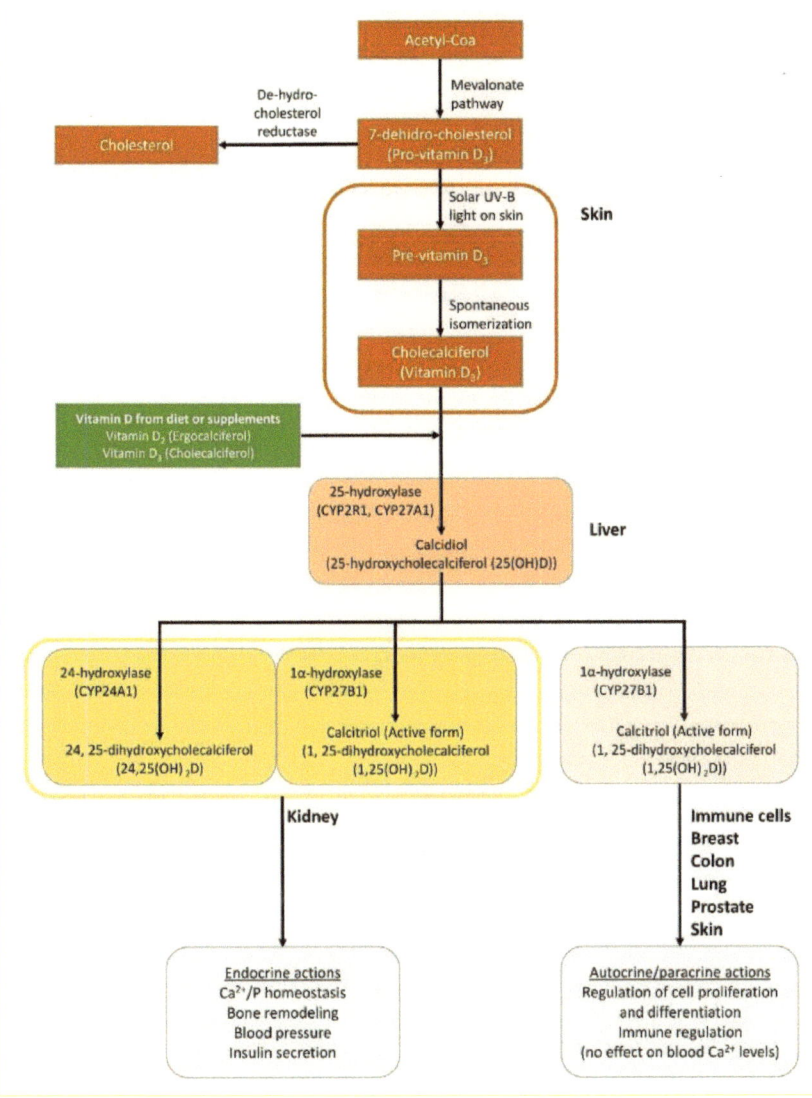

Figure 1: Vitamin D synthesis (8). Vitamin D is synthesised with UV-light energy from 7-dehydro-cholesterol. Cholecalciferol is then metabolised in the liver to calcidiol and activated in various tissues (mainly the kidneys) as calcitriol.

In addition to this long-known part of vitamin D physiology, researchers have recently proven that vitamin D has an immunomodulatory component. Chung et al. discovered that vitamin D levels positively influence tumour angiogenesis and metastasis in breast and colon cancer (9) leading to slower tumour growth and slower disease progression and ivasivity. Manson et al. concluded that cancerous bone health incidents can be partially prevented by oral application of vitamin D, although the exact dosage was not made clear yet (10).

Effects on the Immune System
Vitamin D, specifically 1,25(OH)2D, can bind to the vitamin D receptor that is prevalent in activated B and T lymphocytes, which leads to a decrease in cell activity and the reduced production of IgG and IgM (11). This indicates that vitamin D can actively downregulate an inflammatory immune response towards an anti-inflammatory state by inhibiting the production of pro-inflammatory cytokines such as IL-17 and IL-21 and increasing the production of anti-inflammatory cytokine IL-10. Almerigihi et al. found during an in vitro study that monocytes that are stimulated with CD40 ligands produce fewer interleukins IL-1, IL-6, IL-8, IL-12 and TNFα. Furthermore, they found fewer apoptotic monocytes and, therefore, the decreased release of interleukins into the bloodstream (12). This provokes the hypothesis that vitamin D can be used as a supportive immunomodulator in patients who need immunomodulatory therapy.

Besides B and T lymphocyte interaction, there is also direct interaction with monocytes. Laghishetty et al. found that vitamin D can interact with the CYP27B1 enzyme in monocytes via toll-like receptors, which leads to responses of the innate immunity to exogenous pathogens (13). Other researchers have uncovered evidence that vitamin D can upregulate gene expression in monocytes to increase the secretion of the antibiotic cathelicidin (14). This correlation can even be seen in general monocyte activity outside of infection states: in patients who are vitamin D deficient, levels of cathelicidin are lower than in patients who have sufficient vitamin D levels; the supplementation of vitamin D elevated the patients' cathelicidin levels significantly (15). This implies that higher levels of vitamin D can influence faster innate responses to pathogens and lead to less severe disease courses or even the prevention of symptomatic infection.

Vitamin D and Viral Infections
Taking this supposed immunomodulatory effect into consideration, one could assume that the logical step would be to assess the effectiveness of Vitamin D substitution in patients currently undergoing immune system activation. Some researchers have suggested that the activation of the vitamin D receptor has a broad-spectrum antimicrobial effect by binding 1,25(OH)2D (16). In the following section, vitamin D's influence on different types of viral infections shall be examined.

Vitamin D in upper respiratory tract infections
Upper respiratory tract infections (such as the common cold) are among the highest incidence diseases with 2–3 episodes/a in adults and up to 7 episodes/a in children. Infections are most commonly caused by rhinovirus, coronaviruses and adenoviruses and are characterised by rhinorrhoea, sinusitis, laryngitis and pharyngitis (17). For rhinoviruses specifically, there is only in vitro evidence of vitamin D enhancing the secretion of pro-inflammatory chemokines that lead to a faster and more effective immune response to infection with Human Rhinovirus.

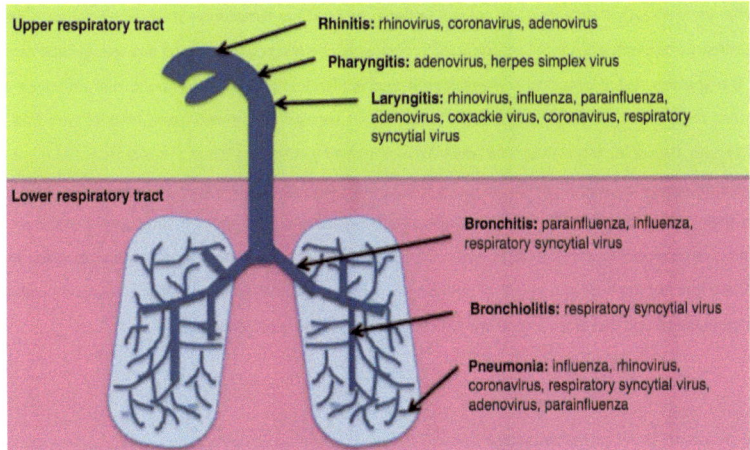

Figure 2: Common viral infections of the respiratory tract (17).

For the upper respiratory tract in general, Jolliffe et al. systematically concluded that an inverse association exists between vitamin D serum levels and the susceptibility to upper respiratory infections. The reviewed clinical trials could, in 50% of the trials, prove a significant reduction in the risk of obtaining an upper respiratory tract infection with a daily intake of at least 300 IU. The daily intake of vitamin D in lower doses, in general, has a better effect than the periodical intake of larger doses of vitamin D (e.g., 100.000 IU/month) (16). The findings from the review conducted by Jolliffe et al. link to the findings of Bryson et al., who found that high levels of 1,25(OH)2D increase the production of antimicrobial peptides such as defensins and cathelicidins while also increasing the expression of TLR and CD14 and macrophage maturation (17).

One could conclude that the regular supplementation of Vitamin D seems to significantly decrease the risk of carrying an upper respiratory tract infection. Therefore, it should be recommended to patients who have a high risk of becoming infected, such as teachers, healthcare staff, populations working in areas with a lot of interaction, etc. after establishing the optimal dosage in clinical trials.

Vitamin D and Influenza

Influenza is a viral disease that is caused by the influenza virus and usually presents with symptoms of an upper respiratory tract infection together with a high, often undulating, fever, myalgia, cephalgia, an unproductive cough and accompanying autonomic symptoms. The treatment of influenza in low-risk patients is usually limited to antipyretics, fluid resuscitation and antitussives. In high-risk patients such as patients who are more than 65 years of age or less than 5 years of age, pregnant women, immunocompromised patients, or patients with a structural lung disease, treatment with antivirals can be indicated as well.

Some researchers have observed seasonal influenza over the last years; the most notable results were published by Cannell et al. in 2006. These researchers described the connection between seasonal influenza and vitamin D levels that were already discovered but not yet understood by Hope-Simpson in 1981. Hope-Simpson was the first scientist to research a potential seasonal influence, which he tracked back to the changes in solar radiation during the seasons. Using historical meteorological and epidemiological data, he found that influenza waves progressed more slowly and produced milder cases when spring and summer were warmer and had more daylight hours. He conducted a study in a small German town by collecting blood samples from the inhabitants over a year to measure 25(OH)D levels. He found them to inversely correlate with the yearly influenza epidemics (18). In their 2008 work, Cannell et al. concluded that considering low infection rates during summer time, Influenza is most probably transmitted by few super spreaders that grow in number during winter when vitamin D levels are low but don't have a vector of infection in summer when vitamin D levels are relatively high in the general population and therefore innate immune responses are more effective (19).

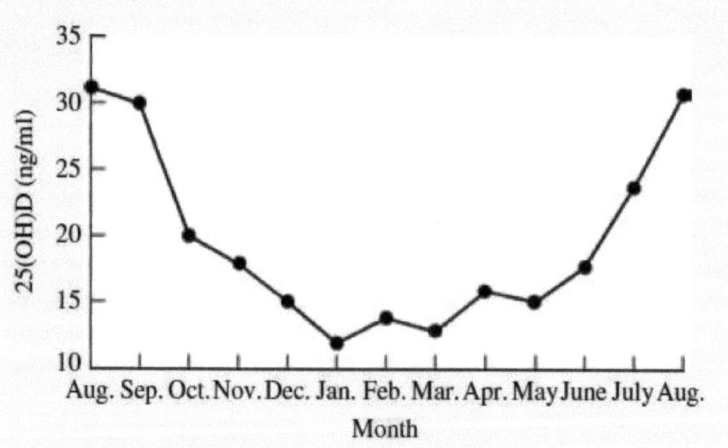

Figure 3: "Seasonal variation of 25(OH)D levels in a population-based sample of inhabitants of a small southern German town, aged 50–80 years."(18) During the months with fewer daylight hours per day, a significant decrease in serum vitamin D levels can be seen. Epidemiological data reveal an increase in upper respiratory infections during this time, which indicates a correlation between those two factors.

Beata Gruber-Bzura notes in her review about vitamin D and influenza that several high-quality studies that were conducted resulted in probands preventively being treated with vitamin D supplements. This led to people being absent from work for fewer days due to respiratory infections and school children having a 42% lower risk of being infected with influenza A according to antibody assays and a lower chance for community-acquired pneumonia-associated comorbidities with higher 25(OH)D serum levels (20).

In 2012 Sundaram et al. found in a review of 10 trials that studied the effects of vitamin D supplementation on respiratory tract infections that no measurable effect on vaccinated groups vs unvaccinated groups could be observed. Furthermore, they generally found lower rates of respiratory tract infections with specifically lower rates for influenza A in Japanese children (21). This implies that the immunity provided by vaccination induced antibody formation and T cell activation is stronger than innate immune reactions as the ones mediated by vitamin D.

Reviewing this data leads to the conclusion that current guidelines for the treatment and prevention of influenza need to be revised, including the evidence from existing clinical trials. Further research is needed when it comes to the exact dosage of vitamin D and relevant cohorts and age groups.

Vitamin D and Herpesviruses

Herpesviridae are common viruses that are prevalent in about 70% of the adult population under 50 years of age. These viruses can be classified into Herpes simplex virus 1 (HSV-1), which causes Herpes labialis and is characterised by small blisters around the lips and the tongue (which are usually being triggered by other infections) (22), and Herpes simplex virus 2, which causes genital herpes and is characterised by genital lesions and scarring. The varicella-zoster virus causes chickenpox, which leads to a fever and a trunk-attenuated exanthema with the possibility to reactivate in later stages of life to cause shingles. The Epstein-Barr virus causes infectious mononucleosis with tonsilitis, lymphadenopathy and fever and is suspected to cause autoimmune diseases such as multiple sclerosis, systemic lupus erythematosus and rheumatoid arthritis. Cytomegalovirus causes a symptom complex similar to that of the Epstein-Barr virus. All herpesviruses have latent phases with periodic reactivation after immune system activation (e.g., shortly after other infections, operations, etc.) (23).

In 2018 Kumar et al. published an in vitro study examining how vitamin D supplementation affects HeLa cells infected with HSV-1. They found that the expression of toll-like receptor 2, which is a pro-inflammatory protein, and the viral titer of HSV-1 were reduced in comparison to a non-supplemented control. They also discovered that supplementation with 1,25(OH)2D was more effective, while supplementation with 25(OH)D had a more persistent effect (24).

For shingles (Herpes zoster), Chao et al. reviewed the connections between vitamin D and the clinical course of herpes zoster. They hypothesised that higher vitamin D levels lower the incidence of herpes zoster in patients. They learned that in a study with immunocompromised dialysis patients, the risk of herpes zoster was significantly lower in patients with vitamin D supplementation, as well as after an infection with the varicella-zoster virus; IgG antibody levels were directly associated with higher serum 25(OH)D levels. They also discovered indirect evidence that vitamin D could benefit patients with postherpetic neuralgia as vitamin D has proven to be effective in patients with diabetic neuropathy, which has a similar pathophysiology to postherpetic neuralgia (25, 26).

Maghzi et al. compared the vitamin D levels of patients infected with the Epstein-Barr virus and an acute episode of infectious mononucleosis to a healthy control group and found a 94,5% higher rate of patients with insufficient vitamin D levels in the group of symptomatic patients than in the control group. The rate of sufficient vitamin D levels was reduced by 66% in the symptomatic group. However, they did not discover any correlations between viral capsid antigen IgM titer and vitamin D levels. They concluded that a low vitamin D level seems to be a risk factor for infectious mononucleosis, whilst mononucleosis itself is a risk factor for autoimmune diseases (27).

The reviewed studies have demonstrated evidence of the positive effect of high serum levels of vitamin D on infections with herpesviruses. Therefore, more high-quality evidence is needed to evaluate which populations benefit the most from the preventive effect of vitamin D and whether it could be used in supportive treatment.

Vitamin D and HIV

Human immunodeficiency viruses (HIV) are a group of viruses known to cause a symptom complex known as acquired immunodeficiency syndrome (AIDS). HIV is caused by a constant depletion of CD4+T lymphocytes over some time (usually 7–10 years), which leads to the immune system's inability to adequately react to infections and causes neoplastic growth.

E. Villamor suggested in 2006 that the serum levels 0f 1,35(OH)2D are often decreased in HIV patients in comparison to the healthy population. He also discovered that mortality rates were higher for HIV patients with lower vitamin D levels. He acknowledged that the evidence is of low quality but provides a trend over several publications (28). Stephensen et al. uncovered no connection between vitamin D serum levels and HIV infections but hypothesised that altered vitamin D metabolism could be a reason for the high prevalence of osteopenia and osteoporosis in HIV patients (29).

J. Lake et al. tried to identify risk factors for HIV patients who have vitamin D deficiency. They claimed that high serum vitamin D levels and high CD4+T lymphocyte counts directly correlate and lead to a slower disease progression. They also suggested that low levels of 25(OH)D in HIV patients are likely to be caused by antiretroviral therapy being administered.

Similarly, Campbell et al. found that in vitro HIV-1 replication could be inhibited by 1,25(OH)D (30). They also learned that macrophage autophagy rates could be increased, which can lead to lower virus titers (31).

Jiménez-Sousa et al. suggested that HIV/AIDS progression could be dependent on serum vitamin D levels as low 25(OH)D levels provoke inflammatory activity and reduce antiviral gene expression via CD4+T lymphocytes, which seem to be less prevalent under low vitamin D levels in general. They also suggested that 25(OH)D may be beneficial in other kinds of immunologic recovery after antiviral therapy (8).

In summary, the evidence for the beneficial effect of Vitamin D on the course of HIV infections towards AIDS seems to be of low quality. It remains unclear whether the recorded benefits are statistical errors due to small sample sizes and inhomogeneous patient groups or actual positive events. This makes more research on the relationship between HIV and Vitamin D inevitable before any recommendations can be provided.

Vitamin D and Viral Hepatitis

Hepatitis viruses A, B, C, D, E and G are a group of viruses comprising different virus families that cause hepatitis of varying levels of severity and after different periods (23). The most common viruses causing hepatitis are A, B and C; therefore, the following analyses will focus on those.

The data on hepatitis A are too limited with only few studies with inhomogeneous sample groups and inconsistent results available to draw any valuable conclusions. Additional clinical data would be needed.

Farnik et al. found in 2013 25(OH)D serum levels and the rate of hepatitis B virus replication correlate. Low levels of vitamin D favour a higher replication rate for viral DNA. The researchers recognised a seasonal pattern that displayed higher viral loads during the winter months and lower viral loads during summer (32).

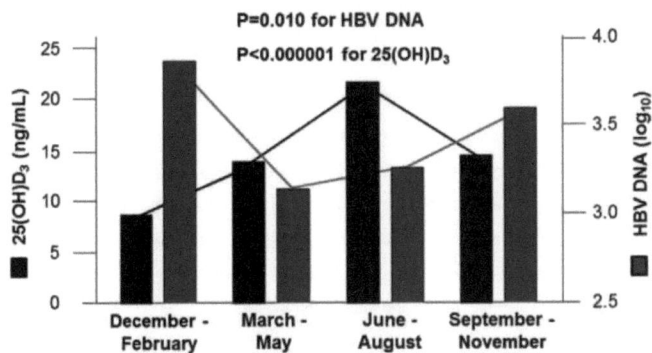

Figure 4: "25(OH)D3 and HBV DNA serum levels are characterised by inversed seasonal variations. 25(OH)D3 and HBV DNA serum levels, measured in the same serum sample, are shown according to season when serum samples were taken for quantification." (32)

In 2016 N. Hoan et al. discovered a correlation between vitamin D status and viral load, as well as disease progression. They found 51,9% of hepatitis B patients were deficient in vitamin D in comparison to 32,5% of the control group. Hepatitis C patients had higher vitamin D levels than hepatitis B patients. In hepatitis B patients, the proportion of deficient patients directly correlated to the disease progression following the Child-Pugh criteria (33, 34). Hoan et al. confirmed Farnik et al.'s assumptions about the association between vitamin D serum status and viral load. The authors suggested that vitamin D be used as an additional part of hepatitis B therapy.

For hepatitis C, researchers have demonstrated through in vitro experiments the antiviral activity of high calcitriol and, therefore, high vitamin D levels in hepatoma cells, which leads to HCV inhibition (35). Additionally, Yano et al. specified a more effective inhibition for higher 1,25(OH)2D levels than for 25(OH)D (36). Rahman and Branch reviewed the data regarding vitamin D and hepatitis C in 2013 and classified vitamin D deficiency as a risk factor for disease progression and adjuvant to improve treatment success. They considered a hepatic influence on vitamin D levels as parts of the hydroxylation process happen in the liver and the supplementation of calcitriol (1,25[OH]2D) was found to be more effective than Calcidiol (25[OH]D) before metabolization (37).

Villar et al. confirmed those findings in a meta-analysis of 11 studies that revealed a rate of 71% for vitamin D deficiency and faster disease progression in patients with lower serum levels. However, they acknowledged that few studies have been conducted on this subject and more studies regarding patients in other geographical areas of the world and ethnicities are needed as it is known that incidences of vitamin D deficiency vary greatly by region (38).

According to the recommendations made by Rahman and Branch, hepatitis C patients with low serum levels of 25(OH)D should receive 2000 IU/day and 2000 IU/d if their levels are below 25 nmol/L (37). More clinical data is needed to determine whether the dosage is adequate and whether there is a difference between the application of Vitamin D2 and D3 regarding vitamin D receptor binding affinity and clinical outcome.

Vitamin D and the Covid-19 Disease

Covid-19

Coronavirus disease 2019 (Covid-19) is a disease caused by severe acute respiratory syndrome coronavirus 2 (SARS-CoV-2). The disease started spreading pandemically in late 2019 and early 2020 and infected around 3,5% of the world population until early December 2021 and caused 5.2 million deaths worldwide. The disease presents with typical symptoms of airway infections such as a fever, cough, headache, fatigue and dyspnoea (39), which are often accompanied by anosmia, ageusia and diarrhoea. Severe cases can develop pneumonia, hypoxia, acute respiratory distress syndrome (ARDS) and multiorgan failure (40).

Covid-19 Pathophysiology

SARS-CoV-2 is a coronavirus that is similar to other respiratory coronaviruses as it enters cells via ciliated pulmonary epithelial cells with a high prevalence of ACE-2 and transmembrane serine protease 2 receptors. The virus is characterised by surface spike proteins that bind to set receptors to activate the process of endocytosis and release the viral RNA genome into the host cell to be replicated by the host's ribosomes. Host driver stones translate the viral polymerase protein to grant the virus full control over the processes in the cell. This leads to further transcription processes for the envelope membrane and surface proteins of SARS-CoV-2, which then leads to the formation of a vesicle around the newly synthesised viral structures and exocytosis of the virus into the body. The high levels of ACE-2 receptors in smokers, obese persons, diabetes patients, cancer patients and other immunocompromised patients offer a potential explanation for the higher rates of severe cases of Covid-19 in those patient groups (41, 42).

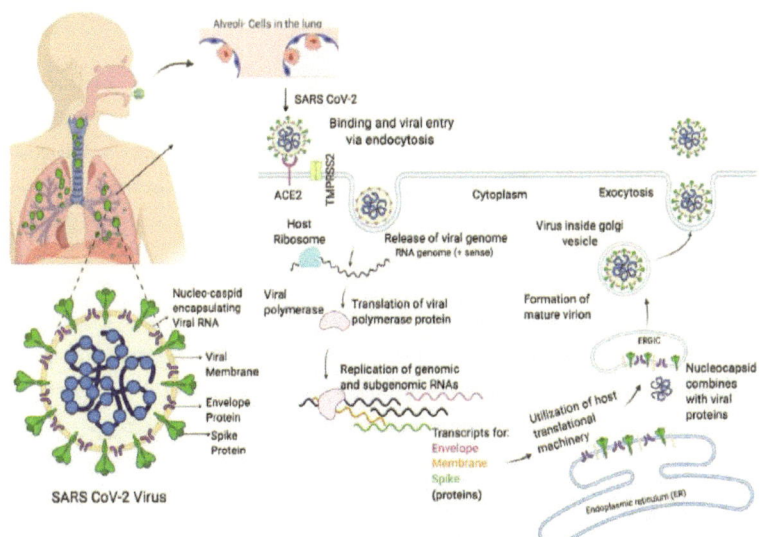

Figure 5: "Molecular drivers of SARS-CoV-2 productive infection" (42). SARS-CoV-2 Virus enters cells via ACE-2 and TMPRSS2 receptors and releases its viral genome into the host cells' cytoplasm. Host cell ribosomes replicate the viral genome and translate into viral organelles. Viral structures are encapsulated and released into the bloodstream or mucosa by exocytosis.

During the first few days after infection, this process of endocytosis, replication and exocytosis repeats continuously in the upper airways. As the viral load continuously grows, the immune system eventually reacts by releasing CXCL-10 and interferons IFN-β and IFN-γ.

The triggering of the immune system leads to the recruitment of macrophages and, therefore, the activation of the adaptive immune system. If the triggered immune reaction is sufficient to keep the viral replication under control, the disease will not progress beyond the stage of an upper respiratory tract infection. Otherwise, the viral load will continue to grow, which can allow the virus to spread to other tissue with a high prevalence of ACE-2 receptors, especially the alveolar epithelial cells in the lungs. This infection of pneumocytes leads to a circulus vitiosus of the continuous infection of healthy lung tissue with viral particles as a result of infected pneumocytes undergoing apoptosis and the release of viral matter due to an immune reaction. This immune reaction is the permanent release of interleukins TNF- α and other reactants, which creates a cytokine storm with an overshooting inflammatory reaction in the interstitial lung tissue (41).

Treatment of the Covid-19 Disease

The current German evidence-based guidelines for treating hospitalised Covid-19 patients by DGINN, DIVI, DGP and DGI recommend maintaining an oxygen saturation of more than 92%. When SpO2 falls below 92% oxygenation using a first nasal cannula, then high-flow oxygen and non-invasive ventilation (CPAP) are considered. If a patient cannot be stabilised and remains in severe hypoxemia (PaO2/FiO2 < 150 mmHg) with respiratory frequencies >30/min, intubation and invasive ventilation are considered. PaO2/FiO2 < 100 mmHg is considered the threshold for required intubation (43).

For pharmacological therapy, patients who are currently on low-flow oxygen receive a combination of dexamethasone with SARS-CoV-2-specific monoclonal antibodies (Casirivimab + Imdevimab). Patients who require high-flow oxygen or NIV therapy should also receive dexamethasone in combination with tocilizumab. Antiviral therapy with remdesivir, which was initially discussed, is no longer recommended. Furthermore, antipyretic therapy, fluid resuscitation and supportive therapy are administered as required by the patient (43).

Prevention of the Covid-19 Disease

To prevent infection with the SARS-CoV-2 virus before vaccinations were available, the most effective measures seemed to be using facial masks of at least medical-grade quality (better than FFP2 or KN95) and maintaining a proper distance from other individuals. Wearing a facial mask does not only protect an individual from viral particles entering their airway but also protects other people by preventing the aerosol generation of the virus by potentially infected but asymptomatic persons. Additionally, regular handwashing and the disinfection of contact surfaces can help prevent infection with SARS-CoV-2 (44).

Since late 2020, several vaccinations against Covid-19 have been made available, including "traditional" vaccines that use an adenovirus as a vector and new types of vaccinations that use mRNA technology. Since the appearance of several new virus variants in 2020 and 2021, mRNA-based vaccines seem to be especially promising in providing immunity against Covid-19. Comirnaty, for example, was found to be effective against infection with a 73% success rate and was effective against hospital admission with a 90% success rate in a study in the United States. Over six months after initial vaccination, effectiveness against infection declined, whilst effectiveness against hospital admission and death remained at over 90% (45).

With the appearance of the new Omicron variant in December 2021, it is unclear whether optimisations of vaccines are necessary as in vitro, the neutralizing activity of antibodies that were formed via vaccination against the new virus variant was very low in comparison to neutralizing activity against the previously dominant Delta variant (Comirnaty: 47% vs. 0%; Spikevax: 50% vs. 0%; Spikevax/Comirnaty: 100% vs. 78%. Preprint data.) (46). It also remains unclear whether vaccines protect against hospitalisation and severe cases of Covid-19 that are caused by the Omicron variant as T cell activity has not yet been studied regarding this variant.

Long Covid and Post-Covid

The prevention of Covid-19 is especially crucial considering that acute infection with SARS-CoV-2 is only one part of the disease. Fifty-seven per cent of Covid-19 survivors develop one or more Long Covid symptoms in the six months after infection. Long Covid symptoms include but are not limited to anosmia, dyspnoea, fatigue, myalgia, headaches, dementia-like symptoms and anxiety (47). The pathophysiology of Long Covid remains unknown to date, but it is suspected that due to the high prevalence of AC-2 receptors throughout cells in the whole body, SARS-CoV-2 can damage more tissue than clinical symptoms would suggest. It is also possible that because Covid-19 possesses some properties of vasculitis, chronic inflammation and autoimmunity continues to pervade affected tissues (48). This hypothesis is backed by researchers who discovered that 52% of Long Covid patients have anti-phospholipid autoantibodies, as well as autoantibodies against interferons, neutrophils, citrulline peptides and nuclei (49).

Currently, there is no causative therapy for Long Covid. As a therapy concept and multimodal therapy including symptomatic therapy are needed, psychotherapy and rehabilitative measures are indicated. It also remains unclear whether it is always possible to differentiate between Long Covid as a new disease and post-intensive care syndrome that has been recognised for a long time.

Dyspnoea needs to be diagnosed via cardiac diagnostic and body plethysmography. In a percentage of patients, pneumological rehabilitation can be indicated.

The best therapy for fatigue involves establishing proper coping mechanisms via psychotherapy after somatic circadian rhythm disorders have been excluded. If chronic fatigue syndrome is suspected, neurologic counselling can be indicated.

In most cases, no therapy is needed to treat anosmia as symptoms resolve within 2–3 months.

Myalgia and headaches often resolve within 2–6 months. During this time, energetic therapy can be indicated; physical therapy and psychosomatic treatment have also proven to relieve symptoms. Anxious patients often also have one or more pain-related symptoms. Anxiety is usually relieved when pain symptoms are relieved (50).

Covid-19 and Vitamin D

As Covid-19 is a disease caused by a coronavirus and is similar to other respiratory infections, a great deal of research has been going on regarding whether the intake of vitamin D has any effect on the prevention, course, or recovery from Covid-19.

In the database clinicaltrials.gov, the search terms "COVID-19", "SARS-CoV-2", and "vitamin D" result in 38 studies marked as completed and 115 studies in general. Using the National Library of Medicine's catalogue PubMed, a search with the same terms results in 935 results. Therefore, the topic can be considered relevant for physicians who are treating patients with Covid-19. Further relevance can be seen for the general population if there were evidence supporting the hypothesis that the supplementation of vitamin D or adequately high vitamin D serum levels would either prevent infection with SARS-CoV-2 or have statistical significance on the outcome.

Bilezikian et al. described an endocrinological concept in which high levels of 1,25(OH)2D might have a protective impact when it comes to the progression of COVID-19 into the RDS phase as it could prevent the "pulmonary cytokine storm". They suggested that calcitriol can decrease dendritic cell activity, which decreases subsequent antigen presentation. Therefore, T cell activation leads to the release of less interference, and other cytokines potentially prevent the disease from progressing. They further suggested that calcitriol can impact cathelicidin production in neutrophil granulocytes, which increases the rate of viral apoptosis (51).

14

Grant et al. confirmed that vitamin D reduces the production of cytokines such as tumour necrosis factor-alpha and interferon γ together with the suppression of T helper cell type 1 activity. The suppression of Th1 cells also reduces the cytokine storm. Furthermore, Grant et al. analysed statistical data and uncovered a correlation between a decrease in the age of 25(OH)D levels and an increase in Covid-19 case fatality rates (52).

Mohan et al. conducted an analysis of statistical data. They discovered that, for example, India, a country with exponential incidence growth during some parts of the pandemic, has a rate of vitamin D deficiency of more than 70% (53).

Borsche et al. compared two meta-analyses against each other; one was based on long-term average vitamin D3 levels in 19 countries, and the other one compared patients who were hospitalised with Covid-19, of which roughly 50% had their vitamin D levels measured after admission and 50% had known vitamin D levels before infection. They found a threshold at 30 ng/ml for a significant decrease of mortality caused by Covid-19. During a linear regression, they also discovered a theoretical threshold of 50 ng/ml at which no mortality would be recorded anymore (54).

Pereira et al. analysed 25 studies that examined the prevalence of vitamin D deficiency in severe cases of Covid-19 disease. They found a 65% higher prevalence of vitamin D deficiency in severe cases of Covid-19 in comparison with mild and moderate cases of Covid-19. They could not confirm whether vitamin D deficiency was already present in the patients before hospitalisation or if it was caused by the disease itself (3).

Taha et al. suggested that the frequent thrombotic events that are caused by Covid-19 15could be a result of vitamin D deficiency. They based their hypothesis on previous evidence that low sun exposure could be a risk factor for deep vein thrombosis together with the fact that the risk of DVT is 50% higher in the winter months (55).

Merzon et al. studied health care workers in Israel for both vitamin D levels and Covid-19 infection. They found that the 10% of their study population (n = 14.022) who had tested positive for Covid-19 at least once on average had a 5% higher rate of vitamin D insufficiency or deficiency. Only 10% of Covid-19-positive patients were vitamin D sufficient with several levels > 30 ng/ml. The mean vitamin D serum concentration in the Covid-19 group was 19 ng/ml, whereas the serum concentration in the Covid-19-negative group was 20.55 ng/ml (56).

Liu et al. discovered that there is a connection between vitamin D serum status and Covid-19 infection and severity. They admitted that the analysed data has a significant publication bias and that it needs to be verified (57).

In summary, it is evident that there is a connection between vitamin D and Covid-19. However, it remains unclear whether the connection is based on Covid-19 interfering with vitamin D or low levels of vitamin D actively causing severe cases of Covid-19 by, for example, upregulating immune reactions that cause a cytokine storm. To determine the connection between Covid-19 and vitamin D, a relevant trial has to be designed. The following section details an example of such a trial.

Study Synopsis

Background

Vitamin D3 (cholecalciferol) is a fat-soluble vitamin that aids in the metabolism of calcium and, therefore, plays an important role in the prevention of rachitis in children and osteomalacia in adults. In recent years, vitamin D has been a part of studies that investigate its impact on the immune system and general health. A meta-analysis published by Zhang Fhang et al. in 2019 suggests that vitamin D supplementation could reduce cancer mortality by 15% (1). An RTC by Shirvani Kalajian et al. (2019) could prove that the expression of certain immune-system-relevant genes changes under different levels of vitamin D (2). Regarding Covid-19, Pereira Damascena et al. proved in November 2020 that amongst hospitalised Covid-19 patients, the rate of vitamin D deficiency was 64% higher than in the mild case group (3). This means that vitamin D supplementation could potentially benefit patients who have Covid-19.

Vitamin D's physiology supports this idea as it is well known that vitamin D's active form, calcitriol (1.25[OH]2D), can modulate the immune system by binding to the vitamin D receptors in various cells and interacting with gene expression and, therefore, cell activity. Vitamin D is known to prevent virally induced ARDS by preventing a cytokine storm (58).

Case reports have revealed that Covid-19 patients have significantly lower serum vitamin D levels than healthy controls (11.1 ng/ml vs. 24.6 ng/ml) (59). It also appears that there is a connection between the severity of vitamin D deficiency and Covid-19 severity as it has been proven that lower vitamin D levels are associated with more severe Covid-19 courses (60).

Researchers have previously found that vitamin D can reduce the risk of developing respiratory tract infections (16). Considering that high-dose supplementations of vitamin D of up to 10.000 international units per day has been established as being safe, different dosages can be studied (61).

Literature research using the terms "vitamin D Covid", "vitamin D Covid-19", "vitamin D Corona" in the PubMed database brought up 15 clinical trials and RCTs; one details the effect of vitamin D supplementation with the reduction of hospitalisations as an outcome. A search in the ClinicalTrials.gov database brought up 115 clinical trials, of which one could be of interest: *The Trial* by Lau et al. uses a combination of Aspirin and vitamin D, which could potentially void gathered data regarding the risk of thromboembolic events as Aspirin is widely used as a thrombocyte aggregation inhibitor. A search for reviews with the same terms brought up (amongst others) a study conducted by Carpagnano et al., who found in 2021 that Covid-19 patients with a 25(OH) vitamin-D level of <10nmol/l had a mortality of 50%, whereas patients with a level of >10nmol/l had a mortality of 5% (58).

Therefore, I suggest supplementing Covid-19 patients with vitamin D to prevent the hospitalisation of individuals who have mild and moderate cases of Covid-19.

Methods

Aims

This study aims to compare the effect of different dosages of vitamin D on four-week hospitalisation rates in patients with mild and moderate Covid-19 cases.

The secondary objectives include the comparison of standard symptomatic Covid-19 therapy following the German guidelines for ambulatory Covid-19 patients versus standard therapy in combination with the supplementation of cholecalciferol without prior serum level measurement in various dosages, as well as the effects of different dosages of vitamin D on the clinical course of Covid-19, both following the WHO's Ordinal Scale for Clinical Improvement (62) and the effect of vitamin D supplementation on the patient-to-patient transmission of SARS-CoV-2 within cohorts.

Design

This study is designed as a randomised control trial with multicentre parallel groups testing for superiority. After the selection of dosage for intervention and the high-dose intervention group, randomisation shall occur using a random number generator to allocate numbers equalling the number of cohorts to all cohorts without considering the time of recruitment. Said numbers shall then be allocated in thirds to the three intervention types. A vitamin D supplement shall be ordered through a local pharmacy and packed according to the cohort progress following the inclusion and exclusion criteria. The cohorts shall be randomised into control and low numbers and shipped to the recruitment centres with the numbers assigned to the cohorts.

Low-Dose Intervention Group

The participants in the low-dose intervention group will receive an initial oral dose of cholecalciferol of 10.000 IU on the day of enrolment into the trial. From Day 2 on, they will receive 1.000 IU/d p.o. for 28 days or until they are excluded from the trial. It is expected that this dosage of vitamin D can increase the serum levels of 25(OH)D by 5–10 ng/ml over the course of the trial. The daily intake of the supplement shall take place during one of the meals at the same time of day for the whole trial. The average daily dose of vitamin D without synthesis and vitamin D taken with food will be 1.321 IU/d, which is below the toxic dose of 10.000 IU/d (61).

High-Dose Intervention Group

The participants in the high-dose intervention group will receive an initial dose of 100.000 IU of cholecalciferol intravenously on the day of enrolment. From Day 2 on, they will receive 5.000 IU/d p.o. for 28 days or until they are excluded from the trial. It is expected that this dosage of vitamin D can increase the serum levels of 25(OH)D by 25–30 ng/ml over the course of the trial. This dosage is a safe dosage that has previously been found to reduce viral replication both in vitro and in vivo (63). The intakes following Day 1 shall be with one of the meals at the same time of day for the whole trial. The average daily dose of vitamin D without synthesis and vitamin D taken with food will be 8.535 IU/d, which is below the toxic dose of 10.000 IU/d (61).

Eligibility criteria

Control group

The participants in the control group shall receive no interventions but will undergo the same monitoring and measurements as the intervention groups.

Inclusion Criteria

Potential participants will be eligible to be included in the trial if their age is above 70 years, they have an active SARS-CoV-2 infection with a positive PCR test that is not older than 48 hours or are isolated together with a SARS-CoV-2 positive patient in the same ward. All the participants must sign an informed consent form to participate in the trial.

Exclusion criteria

Potential participants cannot be included if they do not meet the inclusion criteria, need oxygen therapy, take vitamin D supplements, have contraindications to take any or are currently enrolled in a different clinical trial.

Recruitment process

Potential participating cohorts will be located by actively talking to nursing homes and residential care homes with a ward concept. The nursing homes should be in the same area to eliminate the influence of different strands of SARS-CoV-2 as different disease progressions are endemic in different geographical regions. As soon as a potential cohort is identified, informed consent will be obtained from all ward residents, and randomisation for the event of SARS-CoV-2 infection takes place. As soon as a positive SARS-CoV-2 PCR test for one or more residents is presented and the ward is isolated from its surroundings, interventions will begin for all patients who are willing to participate in the study.

Assessment

All the participants will be asked to provide their health statuses, including any pre-existing conditions, Covid-19 vaccination status and medication plans, which will be anonymised using a standard form on Day 1 and updated with disease-specific treatment data on Days 7, 14 and 28. This data can also be obtained via nurses who are caring for the patients.

Primary outcome measurement

The primary outcome of the study is the hospitalisation rates on Days 7, 14 and 28 within the cohorts. It is expected that even with 100% infection in the cohorts, not all participants will need to be hospitalised for different durations. Measurements that will take place at three points during the trials will account for these variables.

Secondary outcome measurement

The secondary outcomes of the study will be measured by obtaining the OSCI for the patients and comparing them to baseline on Days 7, 14 and 28.

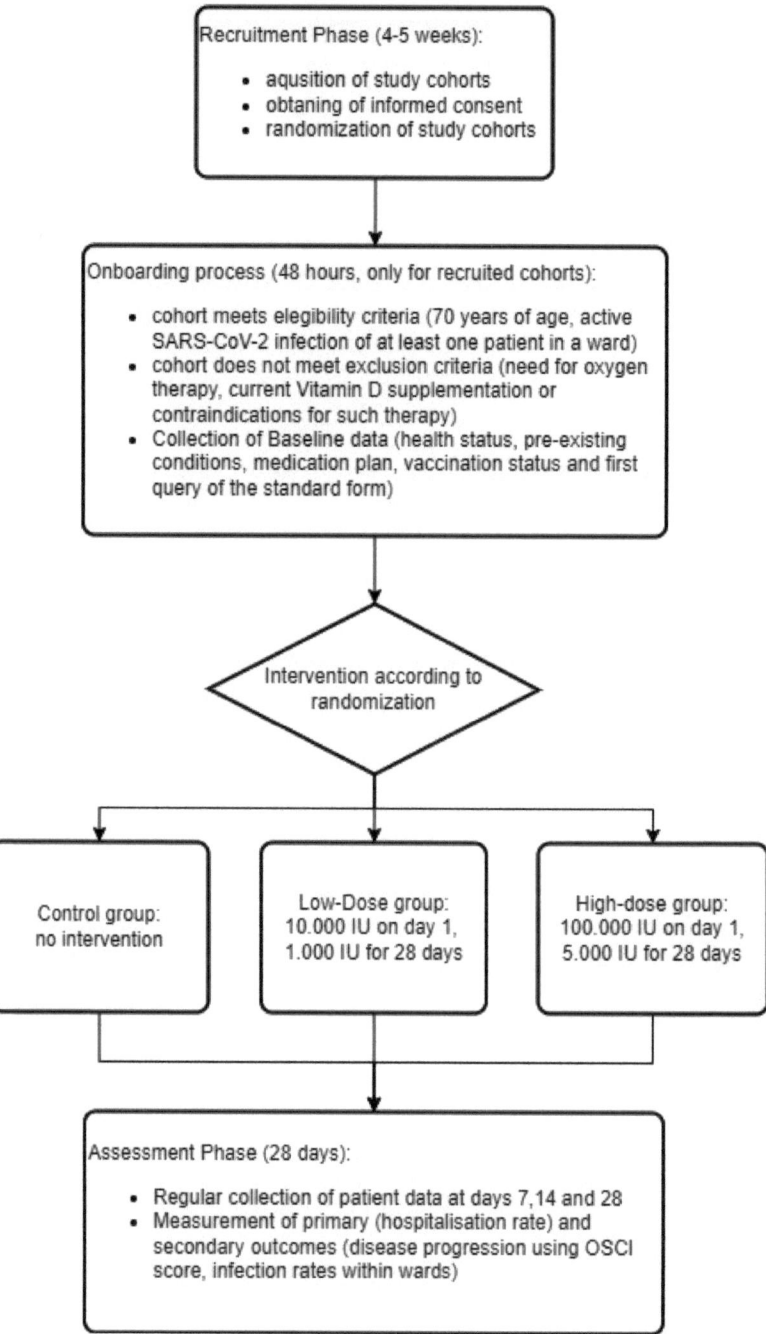

Figure 6: Trial flowchart.

Analyses

Differences between the control and intervention groups will be evaluated using the OSCI scores and the hospitalisation rates on Days 7, 14 and 28 after the trials begin. They will be calculated using descriptive statistical tests, dependence analyses and tests to evaluate tendencies such as the Mann-Whitney test. Hospitalisation rates in the groups will be plotted using the Kaplan-Meier technique.

Ethical considerations

The proposed trial follows the European Medical Agency's guidelines for Good Clinical Practice (64) and the Declaration of Helsinki (65). There are individual benefits for the participants, such as receiving vitamin D supplementation as recommended by the International Association for Gerontology and Geriatrics and potential individual risk reduction of hospitalisation due to Covid-19.

Conclusions

This literature review has provided information that demonstrates that vitamin D seems to have numerous non-skeletal effects that have been only partially studied and even less understood. Previous researchers of Covid-19 have often focused on studying the effects of vitamin D supplementation on mortality or have only descriptively analysed vitamin D status and Covid-19 without intervention. As many countries are currently undergoing the fourth wave of Covid-19 and the Omicron variant's emergence in Europe has led to new exponential growth in incidence, measures to reduce hospitalisation rates and keep intensive care beds free for as many multimorbid high-risk patients as possible are direly needed. Therefore, an interventional study with a widely and cheaply available substance such as vitamin D can assist in finding ways back to normal life without lockdowns and contact restrictions and preserving the limited capacities of healthcare systems worldwide for those who really need them. It should be noted that the vaccinations available against SARS-CoV-2 are safe and effective. If the proposed trial has a positive outcome concerning using vitamin D to reduce Covid-19 hospitalisation rates, it will ever only be supportive of vaccination for elderly high-risk patients who have a physiologically impaired immune system.

Besides potentially being used to combat Covid-19, vitamin D can be used to treat other viral infections such as influenza, upper respiratory infections, or hepatitis as it decreases the viral load and potentially increases phases of immunity with milder cases. On this topic, more research is needed to determine the therapeutic value of vitamin D during active infections as most studies focus on prevention. Having a substance like vitamin D available can be invaluable, especially for countries with lower incomes where expensive medication is not affordable for huge parts of the population. In addition, more knowledge about Vitamin D immunophysiology is needed to completely understand the implications on the immune system. Therefore, it is necessary to study not only elderly patients but, in the future, also larger groups of young patients and to link the results to serum vitamin D levels before any intervention.

Literature Database

Authors, Year	Title	Study type	Sample Size	Results
Jolliffe et al., 2012	Vitamin D in the prevention of acute respiratory infection: Systematic review of clinical studies	Systematic Review	39 Studies	Review of observational studies showed correlations between upper respiratory infections and Vitamin D status, clincal trials were inconclusive.
Bryson et al. 2013	Does vitamin D protect against respiratory viral infections?	Systematic Review	18 Studies	Observational studies found increased risk for upper respiratory infections in patients with lower Vitamin D serum levels, clinical trials were inconclusive.
Gruber-Bzura, 2018	Vitamin D and Influenza— Prevention or Therapy?	Systematic Review	n.a.	Found evidence for decreased risk of upper airway infections for high Vitamin D serum levels. Also studied adverse effects. Found no corellation between Vitamin D levels and Influenza vaccine efficacy.
M. E. Sundaram et al., 2012	Vitamind D and Influenza	Systematic Review	n.a.	Role of Vitamin D in Influenza most probably located in alteration of innate and adaptive immunity, no direct effect on viral activity suspected.
Kumar et al., 2018	25-Hydroxyvitamin D3 and 1,25 Dihydroxyvitamin D3 as an Antiviral and Immunomodulator Against Herpes Simplex Virus-1 Infection in HeLa Cells	Report	n.a.	Supplementation of Herpes Simplex infected Hela cells led to significant decrease in viral activity confirming results of previous studies.
Chao et al., 2014	Serum vitamin D levels are positively associated with varicella zoster immunity in chronic dialysis patients	Report	88 Patients with chronic need for hemodialysis	Serum Vitamin D levels are directly correlated with Varicella Zoster Virus IgG levels suggesting an effect of Vitamin D on long term immunity after infection with Varicella Zoster Virus.
Maghzi et al., 2016	Association Between Acute Infectious Mononucleosis and Vitamin D Deficiency	Case-Control Study	60 Patients, 60 Control	Serum Vitamin D Levels were significantly decreased in Patients infected with Epstein Barr Virus and current acute infectious mononucleosis.
Villamor, 2006	A Potential Role for Vitamin D on HIV Infection?	Systematic Review	n.a.	Vitamin D Levels are significantly reduced in HIV Patients. This is potentially caused by antiretroviral drugs, as in vitro experiments with Human immunodeficiency virus and Vitamin D brought inconclusive results.
Farnik et al., 2013	Low Vitamin D Serum Concentration Is Associated With High Levels of Hepatitis B Virus	Case-Control Study	203 Patients	Inverse correlation between Vitamin D serum levels and Viral

	Replication in Chronically Infected Patients			DNA Serum levels. No estimate of therapeutic value.
Tartof et al., 2021	Effectiveness of mRNA BNT162b2 COVID-19 vaccine up to 6 months in a large integrated health system in the USA: a retrospective cohort study	Retrospective cohort study	3436957 patients	Vaccine effectiveness against Infection with SARS-CoV-2 lowers over a period of 5 months to 47% against delta variant and 67% against other variants. Effectiveness against hospital admission remained high at 93-97%.
Bilezikian et al., 2020	Vitamin D and COVID-19	Systematic Review	n.a.	Vitamin D could be able to supress or attenuate SARS-CoV-2 mediated cytokine storm and therefore prevent ARDS.
Borsche et al., 2021	COVID-19 Mortality Risk Correlates Inversely with Vitamin D3 Status, and a Mortality Rate Close to Zero Could Theoretically Be Achieved at 50 ng/mL 25(OH)D3: Results of a Systematic Review and Meta-Analysis	Meta Analysis	n.a.	Vitamin D serum levels and Covid-19 mortality rate seem to be inversely correlated through several independent patient groups.
Maghbooli et al., 2020	Vitamin D sufficiency, a serum 25-hydroxyvitamin D at least 30 ng/mL reduced risk for adverse clinical outcomes in patients with COVID-19 infection	Retrospective study	235 patients	Significant less patients with a Vitamin D serum level >30 ng/mL had a severe course of COVID-19 disease. Inflammatory markers were inversely correlated with Vitamin D serum levels.

1. Zhang Y, Fang F, Tang J, Jia L, Feng Y, Xu P, et al. Association between vitamin D supplementation and mortality: systematic review and meta-analysis. BMJ. 2019:l4673.

2. Shirvani A, Kalajian TA, Song A, Holick MF. Disassociation of Vitamin D's Calcemic Activity and Non-calcemic Genomic Activity and Individual Responsiveness: A Randomized Controlled Double-Blind Clinical Trial. Scientific Reports. 2019;9(1).

3. Pereira M, Dantas Damascena A, Galvão Azevedo LM, De Almeida Oliveira T, Da Mota Santana J. Vitamin D deficiency aggravates COVID-19: systematic review and meta-analysis. Critical Reviews in Food Science and Nutrition. 2020:1-9.

4. Fleet JC, Schoch RD. Molecular mechanisms for regulation of intestinal calcium absorption by vitamin D and other factors. Critical Reviews in Clinical Laboratory Sciences. 2010;47(4):181-95.

5. Norman AW. From vitamin D to hormone D: fundamentals of the vitamin D endocrine system essential for good health. The American Journal of Clinical Nutrition. 2008;88(2):491S-9S.

6. Bikle DD. Vitamin D metabolism, mechanism of action, and clinical applications. Chem Biol. 2014;21(3):319-29.

7. Lips P. Vitamin D physiology. Progress in Biophysics and Molecular Biology. 2006;92(1):4-8.

8. Jimenez-Sousa MA, Martinez I, Medrano LM, Fernandez-Rodriguez A, Resino S. Vitamin D in Human Immunodeficiency Virus Infection: Influence on Immunity and Disease. Front Immunol. 2018;9:458.

9. Chung M, Lee J, Terasawa T, Lau J, Trikalinos TA. Vitamin D with or without calcium supplementation for prevention of cancer and fractures: an updated meta-analysis for the U.S. Preventive Services Task Force. Ann Intern Med. 2011;2011(Dec.20):827-38.

10. Manson JE, Mayne ST, Clinton SK. Vitamin D and Prevention of Cancer — Ready for Prime Time? The New England Journal of Medicine. 201;364(15):1385-87.

11. Lemire JM, Adams JS, Sakai R, Jordan SC. 1 alpha,25-dihydroxyvitamin D3 suppresses proliferation and immunoglobulin production by normal human peripheral blood mononuclear cells. Journal of Clinical Investigation. 1984;74(2):657-61.

12. Almerighi C, Sinistro A, Cavazza A, Ciaprini C, Rocchi G, Bergamini A. 1Alpha,25-dihydroxyvitamin D3 inhibits CD40L-induced pro-inflammatory and immunomodulatory activity in human monocytes. Cytokine. 2009;45(3):190-7.

13. Lagishetty V, Liu NQ, Hewison M. Vitamin D metabolism and innate immunity. Molecular and Cellular Endocrinology. 2011;347(1-2):97-105.

14. Wang T-T, Nestel FP, Bourdeau V, Nagai Y, Wang Q, Liao J, et al. Cutting Edge: 1,25-Dihydroxyvitamin D3 Is a Direct Inducer of Antimicrobial Peptide Gene Expression. The Journal of Immunology. 2004;173(5):2909-12.

15. Adams JS, Ren S, Liu PT, Chun RF, Lagishetty V, Gombart AF, et al. Vitamin D-Directed Rheostatic Regulation of Monocyte Antibacterial Responses. The Journal of Immunology. 2009;182(7):4289-95.

16. Jolliffe DA, Griffiths CJ, Martineau AR. Vitamin D in the prevention of acute respiratory infection: systematic review of clinical studies. J Steroid Biochem Mol Biol. 2013;136:321-9.

17. Bryson KJ, Nash AA, Norval M. Does vitamin D protect against respiratory viral infections? Epidemiology and Infection. 2014;142(9):1789-801.

18. Cannell JJ, Vieth R, Umhau JC, Holick MF, Grant WB, Madronich S, et al. Epidemic influenza and vitamin D. Epidemiology and Infection. 2006;134(6):1129-40.

19. Cannell JJ, Zasloff M, Garland CF, Scragg R, Giovannucci E. On the epidemiology of influenza. Virol J. 2008;5:29.

20. Gruber–Bzura BM. Vitamin D and Influenza—Prevention or Therapy? International Journal of Molecular Sciences. 2018;19(8):2419.

21. Sundaram ME, Coleman LA. Vitamin D and Influenza. Advances in Nutrition. 2012;3(4):517-25.

22. Opstelten W, Neven AK, Eekhof J. Treatment and prevention of herpes labialis. Canadian Family Physician. 2008;54:1683-7.

23. Ahmad N, Alspaugh JA, Drew WL, Lagunoff M, Pottinger P, Reller LB, et al. Sherris Medical Microbiology. 7 ed: Mc Graw Hill; 2018.

24. Kumar A, Singh MP, Kumar RS, Ratho RK. 25-Hydroxyvitamin D3 and 1,25 Dihydroxyvitamin D3 as an Antiviral and Immunomodulator Against Herpes Simplex Virus-1 Infection in HeLa Cells. Viral Immunol. 2018;31(8):589-93.

25. Chao C-T, Lee S-Y, Yang W-S, Yen C-J, Chiang C-K, Huang J-W, et al. Serum vitamin D levels are positively associated with varicella zoster immunity in chronic dialysis patients. Scientific Reports. 2015;4(1):7371.

26. Chao CT, Chiang CK, Huang JW, Hung KY. Vitamin D is closely linked to the clinical courses of herpes zoster: From pathogenesis to complications. Med Hypotheses. 2015;85(4):452-7.

27. Maghzi H, Ataei B, Khorvash F, Yaran M, Maghzi AH. Association Between Acute Infectious Mononucleosis and Vitamin D Deficiency. Viral Immunol. 2016;29(7):398-400.

28. Villamor E. A Potential Role for Vitamin D on HIV Infection? Nutrition Reviews. 2006;64(5):226-33.

29. Stephensen CB, Marquis GS, Kruzich LA, Douglas SD, Aldrovandi GM, Wilson CM. Vitamin D status in adolescents and young adults with HIV infection. The American Journal of Clinical Nutrition. 2006;83(5):1135-41.

30. Campbell GR, Spector SA. Vitamin D Inhibits Human Immunodeficiency Virus Type 1 and Mycobacterium tuberculosis Infection in Macrophages through the Induction of Autophagy. PLoS Pathogens. 2012;8(5):e1002689.

31. Campbell GR, Spector SA. Hormonally Active Vitamin D3 (1α,25-Dihydroxycholecalciferol) Triggers Autophagy in Human Macrophages That Inhibits HIV-1 Infection. Journal of Biological Chemistry. 2011;286(21):18890-902.

32. Farnik H, Bojunga J, Berger A, Allwinn R, Waidmann O, Kronenberger B, et al. Low vitamin D serum concentration is associated with high levels of hepatitis B virus replication in chronically infected patients. Hepatology. 2013;58(4):1270-6.

33. Hoan NX, Khuyen N, Binh MT, Giang DP, Van Tong H, Hoan PQ, et al. Association of vitamin D deficiency with hepatitis B virus - related liver diseases. BMC Infect Dis. 2016;16(1):507.

34. Hoan NX, Tong HV, Song LH, Meyer CG, Velavan TP. Vitamin D deficiency and hepatitis viruses-associated liver diseases: A literature review. World Journal of Gastroenterology. 2018;24(4):445-60.

35. Gal-Tanamy M, Bachmetov L, Ravid A, Koren R, Erman A, Tur-Kaspa R, et al. Vitamin D: An innate antiviral agent suppressing hepatitis C virus in human hepatocytes. Hepatology. 2011;54(5):1570-9.

36. Yano M, Ikeda M, Abe K-I, Dansako H, Ohkoshi S, Aoyagi Y, et al. Comprehensive Analysis of the Effects of Ordinary Nutrients on Hepatitis C Virus RNA Replication in Cell Culture. Antimicrobial Agents and Chemotherapy. 2007;51(6):2016-27.

37. Rahman AH, Branch AD. Vitamin D for your patients with chronic hepatitis C? Journal of Hepatology. 2013;58(1):184-9.

38. Villar LM. Association between vitamin D and hepatitis C virus infection: A meta-analysis. World Journal of Gastroenterology. 2013;19(35):5917.

39. Islam MA, Kundu S, Alam SS, Hossan T, Kamal MA, Hassan R. Prevalence and characteristics of fever in adult and paediatric patients with coronavirus disease 2019 (COVID-19): A systematic review and meta-analysis of 17515 patients. PLOS ONE. 2021;16(4):e0249788.

40.   Interim Clinical Guidance for Management of Patients with Confirmed Coronavirus Disease (COVID-19): U.S. Centers for Disease Control and Prevention (CDC); 2021 [updated 16.02.2021. Available from: https://www.cdc.gov/ coronavirus/2019-ncov/hcp/clinical-guidance-management-patients.html.

41.   Parasher A. COVID-19: Current understanding of its Pathophysiology, Clinical presentation and Treatment. Postgraduate Medical Journal. 2021;97(1147):312-20.

42.   Chakravarty D, Nair SS, Hammouda N, Ratnani P, Gharib Y, Wagaskar V, et al. Sex differences in SARS-CoV-2 infection rates and the potential link to prostate cancer. Communications Biology. 2020;3(1).

43.   Kluge S, Janssens U, Welte T, Weber-Carstens S, Schälte G, Spinner CD, et al. S3-Leitlinie - Empfehlungen zur stationären Therapie von Patienten mit COVID-19. AWMF online. 2021(113/001).

44.   Bartenschlager PDR, Becker PDS, Brandt PDmC, Dittmer PDU, Eckerle PDI, Liese DmJ, et al. Infektionsprävention durch das Tragen von Masken. AWMF online. (067-010).

45.   Tartof SY, Slezak JM, Fischer H, Hong V, Ackerson BK, Ranasinghe ON, et al. Effectiveness of mRNA BNT162b2 COVID-19 vaccine up to 6 months in a large integrated health system in the USA: a retrospective cohort study. The Lancet. 2021;398(10309):1407-16.

46.   Wilhelm A, Widera M, Grikscheit K, Toptan T, Schenk B, Pallas C, et al. Reduced Neutralization of SARS-CoV-2 Omicron Variant by Vaccine Sera and monoclonal antibodies. 2021.

47.   Taquet M, Dercon Q, Luciano S, Geddes JR, Husain M, Harrison PJ. Incidence, co-occurrence, and evolution of long-COVID features: A 6-month retrospective cohort study of 273,618 survivors of COVID-19. PLOS Medicine. 2021;18(9):e1003773.

48.   Maltezou HC, Pavli A, Tsakris A. Post-COVID Syndrome: An Insight on Its Pathogenesis. Vaccines. 2021;9(5):497.

49.   Zuo Y, Estes SK, Ali RA, Gandhi AA, Yalavarthi S, Shi H, et al. Prothrombotic autoantibodies in serum from patients hospitalized with COVID-19. Science Translational Medicine. 2020;12(570):eabd3876.

50.   Koczulla A, Ankermann T, Behrends U, Berlit P, Böing S, Brinkmann F, et al. S1-Leitlinie Post-COVID/Long-COVID. AWMF online. 2021(020/027).

51.   Bilezikian JP, Bikle D, Hewison M, Lazaretti-Castro M, Formenti AM, Gupta A, et al. MECHANISMS IN ENDOCRINOLOGY: Vitamin D and COVID-19. European Journal of Endocrinology. 2020;183(5):R133-R47.

52.   Grant WB, Lahore H, McDonnell SL, Baggerly CA, French CB, Aliano JL, et al. Evidence that Vitamin D Supplementation Could Reduce Risk of Influenza and COVID-19 Infections and Deaths. Nutrients. 2020;12(4):988.

53.   Mohan M, Cherian JJ, Sharma A. Exploring links between vitamin D deficiency and COVID-19. PLOS Pathogens. 2020;16(9):e1008874.

54.   Borsche L, Glauner B, von Mendel J. COVID-19 Mortality Risk Correlates Inversely with Vitamin D3 Status, and a Mortality Rate Close to Zero Could Theoretically Be Achieved at 50 ng/mL 25(OH)D3: Results of a Systematic Review and Meta-Analysis. Nutrients. 2021;13(10).

55.   Taha R, Abureesh S, Alghamdi S, Hassan RY, Cheikh MM, Bagabir RA, et al. The Relationship Between Vitamin D and Infections Including COVID-19: Any Hopes? Int J Gen Med. 2021;14:3849-70.

56.   Merzon E, Tworowski D, Gorohovski A, Vinker S, Golan Cohen A, Green I, et al. Low plasma 25(OH) vitamin D level is associated with increased risk of COVID-19 infection: an Israeli population-based study. The FEBS Journal. 2020;287(17):3693-702.

57.   Liu N, Sun J, Wang X, Zhang T, Zhao M, Li H. Low vitamin D status is associated with coronavirus disease 2019 outcomes: a systematic review and meta-analysis. International Journal of Infectious Diseases. 2021;104:58-64.

58.   Carpagnano GE, Di Lecce V, Quaranta VN, Zito A, Buonamico E, Capozza E, et al. Vitamin D deficiency as a predictor of poor prognosis in patients with acute respiratory failure due to COVID-19. Journal of Endocrinological Investigation. 2021;44(4):765-71.

59.   D'Avolio A, Avataneo V, Manca A, Cusato J, De Nicolò A, Lucchini R, et al. 25-Hydroxyvitamin D Concentrations Are Lower in Patients with Positive PCR for SARS-CoV-2. Nutrients. 2020;12(5):1359.

60.   Maghbooli Z, Sahraian MA, Ebrahimi M, Pazoki M, Kafan S, Tabriz HM, et al. Vitamin D sufficiency, a serum 25-hydroxyvitamin D at least 30 ng/mL reduced risk for adverse clinical outcomes in patients with COVID-19 infection. PLOS ONE. 2020;15(9):e0239799.

61.   Vieth R. Vitamin D supplementation, 25-hydroxyvitamin D concentrations, and safety. The American Journal of Clinical Nutrition. 1999;69(5):842-56.

62.   Organization WH. WHO R&D Blueprint novel Coronavirus

COVID-19 Therapeutic Trial Synopsis. 2020.

63.   Martínez-Moreno J, Hernandez JC, Urcuqui-Inchima S. Effect of high doses of vitamin D supplementation on dengue virus replication, Toll-like receptor expression, and cytokine profiles on dendritic cells. Molecular and Cellular Biochemistry. 2020;464(1-2):169-80.

64.   Agency EM. Guideline for good clinical practice E6(R2). 2016.

65.   Association WM. WMA DECLARATION OF HELSINKI – ETHICAL PRINCIPLES FOR

MEDICAL RESEARCH INVOLVING HUMAN SUBJECTS. 2013.

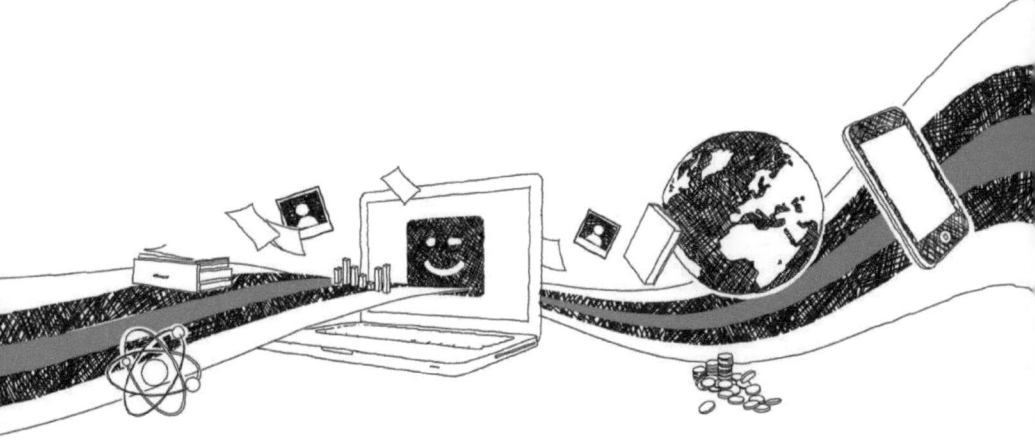
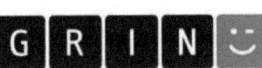